How To Keep Your Dental Fees Way Down And Your Teeth Healthy

343 Great Dental Care Tips That Will Save You Thousands On Dentist Costs

ADAM COLTON

Published by BizMove
www.bizmove.com

Disclaimer

All the content found in this book was created for informational purposes only. The Content is not intended to be a substitute for professional medical advice, diagnosis, or treatment. Always seek the advice of your physician or other qualified health provider with any questions you may have regarding a medical condition. Never disregard professional medical advice or delay in seeking it because of something you have read in this book.

ISBN: 1979382344
ISBN- 978-1979382342

343 Great Dental Care Tips That Will Save You Thousands On Dentist Costs

A healthy mouth is an important part of your overall well-being; gums and teeth can indicate disease long before you're aware that anything is wrong. This book will offer expert advice on keeping your teeth and gums in tip-top shape. Read on for useful information that will keep your smile beautiful.

1. When you start noticing a cavity forming, or any tooth pain, you should call a dentist as soon as possible. This is because once this starts happening, you could lose the tooth. You could also end up spending tons of money getting it replaced. Take care of your teeth regularly and find a dentist in your area.

2. Finding a dentist can be hard especially if you have recently moved into a new neighborhood. There are many websites available that gives dentist scores. You may also find that your primary care physician is a good source for information on dentists located in your community. Additionally, your insurance company may be able to recommend a dentist in your area.

3. How much time do you spend on brushing your teeth? If you want to brush your teeth efficiently,

you will have to spend some time on each tooth so you can brush both sides as well as the space in between teeth. Use an egg-timer if you want to make sure you spend enough time on brushing your teeth.

4. You should always try to brush and floss every day. This time investment will pay off when it comes to your smile. Brushing and flossing is the best preventative maintenance that you can do for your mouth. It's simple, cheap, and doesn't take that much time.

5. Get your children used to brushing their teeth as soon as they start to come in. Wipe infants' teeth clean with a cloth every day so they are used to putting something in their mouth to clean their teeth. When your children become toddlers, let them have a toothbrush to play with and chew on. Then, when they get a little older, show them how to brush their teeth.

6. Make sure you are brushing your teeth two times per day. Don't just brush once. When you sleep, bacteria accumulates in your mouth, so you have to brush first thing in the morning. It is also essential to brush before bed so that you get as much food and bacteria out of your mouth before it goes for hours without being cleaned.

7. Make sure that the toothpaste you use contains fluoride. While there are natural toothpastes available that do not list this as an ingredient, they do not provide the level of protection fluoride does. You have a much higher chance of developing dental issues if you use one of these brands.

8. You can introduce electric toothbrushes to your children starting at the age of three. You should always supervise your children's toothbrushing activities while using these brushes and make sure that your child understands that an electric toothbrush is not a toy and should only be used in his or her mouth.

9. Everyone brushes their teeth, but not everyone brushes their tongues. Whenever you are brushing your teeth it is also important to brush your tongue as well. There are several different bacteria that thrive on your tongue so make sure you keep your entire mouth clean by scrubbing your tongue too.

10. If you're doing teeth whitening, stay away from foods and drinks that stain teeth. These foods can make any teeth whitening efforts to fail. Keep your new smile shining bright by changing your habits.

11.　　Sometimes in life we have to make decisions about our health. For example, we may want to eat right, but we don't have time for a healthy restaurant. Instead, we choose a salad at a fast-food joint. The same can be said of dental care - for example, mint floss is a great way to convince yourself to floss more often.

12.　　Keep an eye on your gums, and take note of any decay. This is the most vulnerable part of teeth, as it's right where the nerves begin. Gingivitis is a common disease of the gums, due to poor oral hygiene. Watch this area carefully and call your doctor if you notice any visible changes or pain.

13.　　If you have been putting off going to the dentist because you are afraid of what they may find, don't put it off another day. Tooth problems do not fix themselves. You have to go eventually. If you are afraid of the dentist look for one that offers sedation so that you sleep through the entire visit.

14.　　Do you have a habit of opening plastic packages and bottles with your teeth? Don't ever do this again! This can cause permanent damage to your teeth. Additionally, there is a high likelihood of bacteria being present.

15.   Replace your toothbrush every three months. Even if you are extremely dedicated to cleaning your toothbrush properly, it's best to safe and not play chances with bacteria. Plus, bristles wear down after months of usage, so they don't clean as well. This goes whether you have an old-fashioned tooth brush or an automatic brush with cleaning heads.

16.   Change your toothbrush every few months. If you have an electric toothbrush, change the head on it. An old toothbrush can collect bacteria and when you brush you are putting that into your mouth. Be safe and avoid the bacteria by changing it every 2 months for a healthier mouth.

17.   There are many common foods and drinks which cause your teeth to look stained. Wine, tea and coffee are common beverages which stain the teeth. Colas and gravies do as well. You do not have to avoid these foods and drinks, but you should remember to brush and floss as soon as possible after eating or drinking them.

18.   Teeth and gums say a lot about a person's health. Of course you want to have the best looking set of teeth possible but it's important to go beyond that and understand the implications of oral problems and what you can do about them. Keep

your smile bright and healthy for a long time to come!

19.   Don't wait to see a dentist. If you've started feeling even the slightest bit of pain in your teeth, make an appointment with a dentist. If you wait too long the problem could get even worse. If you get in right away, you may only need a quick and easy treatment.

20.   Fluoride can be a great ally in the fight to maintain a healthy smile and strong teeth. If your household water is not fluoridated, everyone in your home may have problems with tooth decay. One thing you should do is to be sure that fluoride is in your toothpaste. Another possible option is using a mouthwash or rinse that contains fluoride.

21.   For truly clean teeth, pick a toothbrush that has soft bristles that is adequately sized for your mouth. Let your brush dry in the air to avoid bacteria growth. Keep it upright and in a place where the air circulates.

22.   Remember that you are what you eat, and so are your teeth. If you smoke a lot and drink red wine often, your teeth do get discolored. If you want whiter teeth, change what you eat. If it's dark going

on your mouth, your teeth are going to get dark from it.

23.   Schedule a visit to your dentist if you have sensitive teeth. Pain in your teeth when eating hot foods or drinking cold drinks may be indicative of serious dental issues. You may have a cavity, nerve inflammation, or nerve irritation. These are dental problems you do not want to ignore.

24.   It is important to make things fun when teaching young children how to care for their teeth. Let them pick out their own kid-friendly tooth paste and tooth brush so that they will be excited about using it. Children tend to respond better when you actually offer them choices and allow them to make their own dental care decisions, within reason.

25.   Your daily mouthwash should be natural and alcohol free. These formulations burn your mouth less, and also help if you suffer from halitosis. The alcoholic mouth washes can give you an hour or two of minty-fresh breath, you can also end up with a dry mouth. Dry mouth then leads to bad breath.

26.   While mint is one of the most popular flavors for toothpaste, if you don't like it, you must find a flavor you do like. Toothpaste is available in numerous flavors besides the standard mint. Pick

up a product with a favorite flavor, as this will make it easier to tolerate. You may also be able to special order different flavors from a holistic store or pharmacy.

27.   Finding a good dentist is important, but it is equally important to practice good oral hygiene every day. Make sure to brush your teeth in the morning and evening. Use a soft-bristled, gentle toothbrush, and brush all surfaces of each tooth. Doing this will help to keep your teeth healthy in between dental visits.

28.   Always look to healthy snacks to lower the amount of junk foods in your diet that can harm your teeth. When you don't, brush your teeth soon to rid your mouth of excess sugar. This will reduce the chance of getting cavities.

29.   If you have gum disease, you should postpone any plans to undergo cosmetic dental procedures. For the best results, your teeth and gums must be healthy. Otherwise, you will be more prone to infections, or may need to repeat the procedure. Avoid any dentist who is willing to take a chance on your health by risking this.

30.   Talk to your dentist about what kind of toothpaste you should use. Your dentist has a

knowledge base to know what is good and what is just fancy packaging. Not only that, but your dentist can consider your particular teeth and choose one that works best for you and your lifestyle.

31.   Before shelling out thousands of dollars for veneers, think about your reason for wanting to do so. Is your only goal to have whiter teeth? If so, skip the veneers in favor of bleaching or other whitening procedures. While veneers will allow you to have whiter teeth, they are best used on patients who want to make their teeth appear longer.

32.   Brush your tongue. Your tongue needs attention just like your teeth and gums do. Use your toothbrush and brush your tongue just like you brush your teeth. Not only is this good for your dental health, but it can help with any bad breath you may be experiencing, too.

33.   When you want to eat something between meals, try to avoid sugary snacks. These will just leave your teeth open to cavities and decay. Instead, have fruit or vegetables, or even whole grain carbohydrates. These are better for your overall health as well as your dental situation, but don't forget to brush after!

34. Think about switching up to an electronic toothbrush if you have not already. These devices are increasingly recommended by dental professionals. The reason for this is the strong performance they offer compared to manual brushing. Electric toothbrushes are able to cup around teeth and work faster. They also do a better job of cleaning the specific sites that bacteria and plaque tend to accumulate in.

35. Don't settle for using just any toothpaste. This is when it's time to buy expensive. Buy a product that has baking soda or a whitening formula and one that fights against tartar and plaque. If need be, get a recommendation from your dentist, and this will make your mouth feel instantly better.

36. What kind of toothpaste do you use? It is best to use a toothpaste that contains fluoride. If you have issues with cavities, choose a toothpaste designed to reduce your risks of developing cavities. You can also choose a product designed for people with sensitive gums if this is your case.

37. Eat what are known as detergent foods. These are foods that naturally clean your mouth as you eat them. Apples are the most famous example. Other choices include raw carrots, celery and popcorn.

Ending a meal with a detergent food is a great way for your mouth to end the eating cleaner.

38.   One of the things that you will need to make sure to do when you are taking care of your teeth is to floss. This is very important as it will help to get rid of the excess food between your teeth that your toothbrush cannot reach. This will lead to better overall health.

39.   A healthy diet is one of the best things you can do to make sure your teeth stay health. Avoiding sugary drinks and foods is important to avoid harming the enamel of your teeth. Fresh fruits and vegetables are the best choice when it comes to promoting healthy teeth and gums.

40.   You may have a lot on your plate with work and home, but you should reserve time for proper dental care. The time you spend on this is something that will pay off later on. Nothing protects your mouth like brushing and flossing your teeth. It's inexpensive, easy, and necessary in order to have a dazzling smile.

41.   Brush ALL of your teeth, every single time. The act of brushing your teeth seems simple enough, so why do so many people do it incorrectly. A recent survey of dentists reveals that one of the most

common mistakes people make is brushing only their front teeth. Don't focus on brushing only the teeth that other people see. Your molars and other back teeth are equally important, so don't neglect them!

42.   Disclosing tablets and mouthwashes can help you identify potential plaque build-up on your teeth. Prior to brushing, swish or chew the product in accordance with package directions. The blue or pink stain will highlight any areas with buildup. It can be time consuming to brush all the dye away, so make sure you have adequate time available. Definitely not a great idea if you are in a rush to get somewhere!

43.   Strengthen your existing enamel with the foods that you eat. Certain vitamins and the mineral calcium, in particular, all help out with this. Foods that are good to accomplish this with include nuts, meats and dairy choices. Avoid sugary foods, soft drinks and sweetened teas, as these will do immediate damage to your enamel.

44.   As you floss, focus on just one tooth before turning your attention to the next one. Work the floss down to your gum line and then carefully pull it back up to get rid of any plaque that has

accumulated. In a back-and-forth motion, rub the floss so that it cleans the tooth well.

45.   You need to visit the dentist twice a year for a check-up and cleaning to keep your mouth in tip-top shape. The cost is worth it when you consider how much you will be billed when you have to have a cavity filled, root canal or extraction! Don't forget the cost of dentures!

46.   Before you choose a dentist, check to see if they are a member of the American Dental Association. This group is abbreviated as the ADA. There are professional standards that are the same nationwide for an oral hygiene professional to join. You can also just visit the ADA website to start your local dentist search.

47.   When flossing, don't be skimpy on the amount of floss you use. Use a piece around eighteen inches in length. When you use too little floss, you'll often lose your grip on the floss itself. Then it becomes an aggravating experience that you aren't likely to make into a habit.

48.   When choosing a toothpaste, make sure that the product you choose includes fluoride. You can choose any flavor or brand you prefer, or you can even choose paste or gel. In fact, there are great

kids options on the market which have glitter in them! That'll convince them to brush!

49.   If you think you may have a dental problem, don't wait too long to visit the dentist. If you have issues like cavities, see a dentist right away. If you delay going, that cavity can worsen. Instead of getting a filling, you may need to have a root canal.

50.   Avoid eating sticky sweets that may get stuck between your teeth and hard foods that can crack them. Smoking and drinking certain beverages, like red wine and coffee can stain your teeth. Eat a high calcium diet and get an adequate amount of Vitamin C. Crunchy fruits and vegetables can clean your teeth naturally.

51.   If you aren't going to be brushing right after your meals, close your meal with hard foods that protect your teeth. Good foods for your teeth include apples, celery and carrots. These foods can help clean your teeth.

52.   If you've got stained teeth, try gargling with a little apple cider vinegar before brushing your teeth. The vinegar will kill off pesky bacteria and actually help clean those stains over time. Doing it right before brushing is especially beneficial as it'll

increase the stain removal potential. It's a great one-two punch!

53.   In order to maximize the effectiveness of brushing, be sure to keep the toothbrush at the correct angle. The brush should be held at a 45 degree from the gum line. This angle allows the brush to reach up into the areas between the gum line and the teeth. Plaque tends to accumulate in these areas, and using the proper angle can help minimize this.

54.   If you frequently experience dry mouth and bad breath, you probably feel embarrassed or self-conscious when you speak with others. To remedy this problem, treat yourself to a piece of gum or hard candy that contains xylitol. You can also use a scraper or soft-bristled toothbrush to gently clean the top, underside and end of your tongue once or twice daily.

55.   A healthy diet is one of the best things you can do to make sure your teeth stay health. Avoiding sugary drinks and foods is important to avoid harming the enamel of your teeth. Fresh fruits and vegetables are the best choice when it comes to promoting healthy teeth and gums.

56.   Ask your friends and family for dentist referrals. They can really be your greatest resource for having questions you are curious about answered honestly. Also, they can inform you of how much they charge, which is particularly useful if you are on a budget.

57.   If you would like your teeth to be healthier, consume more dairy products. Cheese, yogurt and milk all contain the calcium you need. Use calcium supplements if you cannot eat dairy. It wont be long until you find that your teeth seem whiter and you have fewer cavities.

58.   Take your time when you brush. Brushing for a minute or less is not enough time to thoroughly clean your mouth. It is recommended that you brush for at least two minutes every time you brush, but three minutes is also fine. Anything over that is too long and can be counterproductive to your oral health.

59.   Sometimes eating certain foods is helpful after you've had a meal. In fact, eating an apple after a meal can help loosen debris from the teeth and gums and get your mouth feeling fresh again. It also can remove built up gunk from the surfaces of your teeth, plus it's low in sugar.

60.   When it comes to taking care of your teeth, the best thing, you can do is brush your teeth twice a day. Most of us are good about brushing each morning, but not nearly as many people choose to brush at night. When you don't brush your teeth at night, you are allowing all the bacteria you've collected throughout the day to breed throughout the night.

61.   Replace your toothbrush every three months. The bristles on your toothbrush, no matter how much you clean them, wear out over time. They lose their cleaning effectiveness after a few months. Do yourself (and your mouth) a favor and have a replacement handy when you hit that 90 day mark.

62.   You should replace your toothbrush every three months. As you use a toothbrush, the bristles wear out. When the bristles become worn, your toothbrush can harm your gums. This can cause your gums to begin bleeding. For best results, choose a toothbrush with a small head and soft bristles.

63.   When brushing your teeth, avoid always starting in the same place. If you always start in the same place, you will typically do a very good job in that place, and a not so great job as you get to the end of your brushing section. To avoid skimping on

sections of your mouth, change up your starting position.

64.   Use mouthwash after you brush. Mouthwash contains anti-bacterial properties that help prevent the build-up of plaque. After you brush, swish a mouthful of mouthwash around your mouth to rinse your teeth and gums. You can also use mouthwash in the morning after you get up to eliminate your morning breath.

65.   Use apple cider vinegar as a mouthwash in the morning. This is an excellent way for you to get fresh breath, but more than that, apple cider vinegar can also get rid of stains on your teeth and make your teeth appear brighter. Apple cider vinegar is very inexpensive, so this is a wonderful tool in your dental care.

66.   The newest thing in candy is sour flavored candies. But these candies contain a high level of acid and sugar which is a perfect combination to erode the enamel and cause cavities. You should avoid such candies if you can, but if you or your children eat them, then rinse your mouth afterwards.

67.   Keep a close eye on the health of your mouth. You are the one that lives with your mouth and are

most able to realize that something is not right. If you notice any pain or swelling you should seek the advice of your dentist as soon as you can.

68.   To make sure you get the most out of brushing, make sure that you don't eat any food after you brush for the night. If you are thirsty, you can drink some water. However, food or drinks with any sugar will leave a residue on your teeth overnight, undoing much of the work you did by brushing.

69.   Although the majority of people use teeth whitening products without experiencing any negative consequences, there are some possible side effects you should be aware of. Exposing the dentin layer to certain teeth whitening chemicals can increase tooth sensitivity. Whitening solutions can also cause chemical burns may lead to gum irritation and redness.

70.   When it comes to creating strong, healthy teeth, fluoride can be your best friend. If fluoride is not added to your public water supply, you will be more susceptible to tooth decay. One choise is to brush with a toothpaste that contains it. A mouthwash rich in fluoride is another good option.

71.   Do not forget to remove plaque from your teeth when flossing. You should place the floss at the

bottom of the tooth and gently pull it so it scrapes the plaque off your tooth. Do this for each tooth before focusing on cleaning the space between your teeth with floss.

72.   Examine your toothbrush several times a month. Look for signs that you might need to buy a new one. The bristles are often the first indication. If you see that they are becoming frayed, go out and purchase something else. In general, you shouldn't go longer than four months without getting another brush.

73.   Your daily dental hygiene regimen is not complete unless you floss at least once a day. You need also make certain that you are using a proper technique. Gently slide it between the teeth you wish to clean. Move the floss backwards and forwards. Don't allow your floss to slide under your gums. Instead, keep it at your gum line. Clean your teeth with the floss, one-by-one.

74.   Be realistic about your expectations for whitening toothpastes. The compounds and abrasives they contain are often very helpful at lightening the surface stains on your teeth, such as coffee stains. However, they are not going to address more serious issues like decay or stains that have penetrated the tooth enamel. Most dental

experts agree that it is safe to use such toothpastes twice a day.

75.   When putting your baby to bed, do not allow them to keep a bottle in their mouths that contain juice or milk. This will cause the sugars in the liquid to settle on the teeth, which can cause all of their teeth to rot. If you must give them a bottle, it should be filled with plain water.

76.   Consider purchasing electric toothbrushes for the whole family. They cut down the effort you have to produce to get the same results with a manual brush. Electric toothbrushes are not only affordable, but are recommended by most professional dentists. They have solid bristles which cup around your tooth and quickly help brush away plaque.

77.   Smoking can wreak havoc on gums and teeth. If you currently see no damage, just look up some information and images about the damage smoking can do to your mouth, teeth and gums. Make an effort to quit smoking as soon as possible. Speak with a doctor or a dentist about what you can do to stop now.

78.   The time you spend brushing your teeth should never be less than a full two minutes. The longer

you brush, the more debris you can get rid of. If you do not brush long enough, you will not to a good job, and could end up with decay.

79.   Mouthwash is important in dental hygiene. Mouthwash can rinse out the areas of your mouth that are not able to be reached by a toothbrush. Rinse once each morning and once each night. Pick a non-alcohol mouthwash, as alcohol is drying to the mouth.

80.   If you are having a difficult time paying for necessary dental work, consider visiting a dental college. College students in the later stages of their training need real people to work on, and they will often perform work at a significantly reduced cost. All students are supervised by their professors or certified dentists, so you remain in safe hands during your procedure.

81.   Do you tend to grind your teeth? Do your best to get rid of this habit. Avoid eating hard foods, chew some gum and relax as much as you can. If you grind your teeth at night, it is best to wear a mouth guard until this bad habit goes away.

82.   Regardless of your age, brush your teeth at least twice a day. Use a soft bristled toothbrush and replace it every couple of months, or whenever the

bristles become worn out. Do prevent decay and strengthen your teeth, use fluoride toothpaste, rinse with a fluoride mouth wash and floss every day.

83.   If one or more of your teeth is in pain, avoid placing aspirin right next to them. It is an old wive's tale that an aspirin next to the tooth will dissolve the pain. This can actually cause it to burn and decay.

84.   Be sure to get any chips or cracks in your teeth as soon as possible. When you have a cracked or chipped tooth, you are giving germs and bacteria a great place to hide. Obviously, when you have these problems fixed, bacteria and germs have nowhere to go. Fluoride mouthwash can also help.

85.   Change your toothbrush every few months. If you have an electric toothbrush, change the head on it. An old toothbrush can collect bacteria and when you brush you are putting that into your mouth. Be safe and avoid the bacteria by changing it every 2 months for a healthier mouth.

86.   There are a number of over-the-counter teeth whitening products. They can make your smile look dazzling. But you also need to floss, brush and see the dentist regularly. Your teeth can look superficially white while you are suffering from gum

disease or cavities. Teeth whitening is no substitute for proper dental care.

87.   If you've ever wondered if there was a way to make it easier on yourself to take care of your mouth, then you need to keep reading. There are many tips and tricks available, from selecting the right toothpaste to choosing the right dentist. Keep reading to find out more about making your job easier.

88.   You may already know that you have to brush your teeth a couple times a day if you wish for them to be as healthy as possible. You may not know that there are some times when you must brush more frequently, however. You can keep your enamel in good shape and prevent cavities by brushing any time you have high sugar food or drink.

89.   How you move your toothbrush can directly influence how well it will clean your teeth. While brushing, hold the brush at an angle rather than straight. Then, move it around in circular fashion. Don't brush too hard as that will agitate your gums.

90.   If sparkling white teeth from a toothpaste sounds too good to be true, that's because it is. While non-prescription whitening pastes and rinses may remove light stains on the surface of teeth, they

will not produce the best possible results. Only your dentist can help you to achieve these results, often with bleach.

91.   You ought to choose healthy foods when you can, to avoid teeth damage. If you must have sugar-laden snacks, be sure to finish them fast and brush your teeth immediately. This reduces the chance of cavity growth.

92.   If your dentist tells you that you need to have a tooth out or that you have to take antibiotics, follow his or her directions. Get the pills or get the tooth removed as soon as you can after your initial appointment. Oral infections can spread quickly to other parts of your body if they are not dealt with immediately. This is why it is so important to address infections promptly.

93.   Do not continue to see a dentist with whom you do not feel right. Your dental health should be a priority. Do not hesitate to switch to a different dentist if you are not satisfied with your current care provider.

94.   Do you like chewing ice? If so, stop it immediately. You can crack your teeth by chewing on ice, and the cold temperature can make the sensitive nerves feel very painful. Try chewing on

sugarless gum instead. If needed, do not put any ice cubes in your drinks. Otherwise, you may be tempted to munch away.

95.   Sugar feeds the bad bacteria found in your mouth. To help avoid feeding the bacteria brush your teeth immediately after consuming a sugary drink or food. To help protect your mouth and increase the beneficial bacteria found in your mouth take a probiotic supplement daily. Use both methods to increase the health of your mouth.

96.   Make sure you change your toothbrush once every two or three months. After a few months of use, your toothbrush's bristles will wear out and will no longer effectively brush. This same rule applies for electric toothbrush heads. If your toothbrush is wearing out before two months, it could be a sign that you're brushing your teeth too harsh.

97.   Drink soda and non-water beverages with a straw. That helps them to avoid contact with your teeth. That will help keep your teeth clean, but it will also keep them white. If you cannot use a straw, make sure you brush as soon as you can after drinking those things.

98.   You can remove 99% more plaque from your teeth by using oral irrigators. Try using this device

instead of flossing, as it is more effective. These device use pressurized water streams to get between your teeth where brushing alone can't reach. Your chances of optimal gum health are also increased by 93% using this device.

99. A regular toothbrush must be replaced frequently. Electric toothbrushes need heads rotated frequently. Using the same brush for months or even years can just transfer bacteria back into your mouth. You should change your toothbrush every couple of months.

100. Make time to clean your tongue every time that you brush your teeth. Your tongue can hold a lot of germs and needs to be kept as clean as possible. A clean tongue also promotes fresh breath. If you want to do everything you can to have a healthy mouth you will follow this tip regularly.

101. When choosing a toothpaste, make sure that the product you choose includes fluoride. You can choose any flavor or brand you prefer, or you can even choose paste or gel. In fact, there are great kids options on the market which have glitter in them! That'll convince them to brush!

102. If you are not brushing for at least two minutes, you should try to increase your brushing time. In

order to do this, you can separate your mouth into four sections, such as your top teeth on your right side. Start brushing in one section, and continue until 30 seconds are up. Once the 30 seconds are up, move onto the next section.

103.   Avoid food and beverages that are high in acid unless you can brush immediately after consuming them. Drink soda, tea and coffee through a straw whenever possible to limit contact. Brush your teeth or rinse your mouth with water immediately after eating citrus fruits, tomatoes and other acidic fruits.

104.   Use an electric toothbrush to brush. An electric toothbrush moves the brush head at a greater speed than what you can achieve when using a manual brush. The additional movement of the brush head cleans your teeth more effectively and with less effort. You can use your manual toothbrush when you brush between meals when not at home.

105.   If you're having a problem with a tooth infection and you can't make it to the dentist, try the emergency room. An infection can do a lot of damage to your body if it goes untreated. You will get antibiotics but it will cost you quite a bit of money.

106.   If even a tiny amount of blood is present when you brush your teeth, make an appointment to meet with your dentist. Don't ignore the most common sign of gum disease -- bleeding, painful gums. This can make you lose your teeth and get infections.

107.   Make sure you floss. While brushing is a good habit, it isn't enough to protect your teeth. Food particles often lodge between the teeth; this can lead to tooth decay if not addressed immediately. Flossing after every meal can help remove debris from between the teeth so that you can ensure optimal dental health.

108.   Are you hit with a sudden pain sensation when your teeth come in contact with hot or cold foods or drinks? Use toothpaste that is made for extra-sensitive teeth or gums. Then visit the dentist at your earliest convenience. Sensitivity might be a sign of a cavity or nerve inflammation. You need to get these problems treated right away.

109.   When choosing a dentist, don't forget to think about location. Do you work? Would it be more convenient to go to someone who is near your office? Or would you prefer to go to someone that is close to your house? If it is inconvenient to get to your dentist, you might not go, which is why it is important to consider this factor.

110.   Flossing picks are a great tool if you have trouble flossing. A flossing pick has a string that is connected by two pieces of plastic. They are convenient to use virtually anywhere. You might forget to floss, but some find these sticks easier to remember. The flossing picks can also be a training aid for children.

111.   If you want your teeth to stay healthy and you enjoy having a beautiful smile, you should see your dentist every six months. Getting your teeth cleaned twice per year will help them to stay clean and free of unsightly tartar and plaque build up. Regular dental checkups are the key to preventing dental decay.

112.   Drink three glasses of milk a day for a healthy smile. Milk is high in calcium, which your teeth need, and it can also help to keep your teeth white. If you want to have the brightest, healthiest smile around you will be sure to drink your three eight ounce servings of milk every single day.

113.   Keep your mouth clean and healthy by replacing your toothbrush every other month. Your best bet is to choose a soft- or medium-bristled toothbrush. Harder brushes could potentially erode the enamel or cause your gums to bleed. Purchase a name-

brand brush so that you are assured the quality is good.

114.   Even if you're an adult, it's never too late to get braces. It's important to have a smile which looks good and keeps you happy, so it's worth it to invest the time and money into getting the straightest teeth possible. This can open doors both socially and professionally, so consider it for yourself.

115.   Many people with bad breath are missing one important part of their oral hygiene process - brushing their tongue! In fact, just by brushing their tongue, people find that they quickly fix their problem and end up with fresh, clean breath in no time, so give it a try yourself!

116.   When choosing a toothpaste, make sure that the product you choose includes fluoride. You can choose any flavor or brand you prefer, or you can even choose paste or gel. In fact, there are great kids options on the market which have glitter in them! That'll convince them to brush!

117.   The first mistake that people make in dental care is to buy the wrong toothbrush. You should choose a toothbrush that fits well in your mouth and reaches all areas. Your toothbrush should also fit

well in your hand. If you lose your grip on your toothbrush, you could actually injure yourself.

118.   Bleeding gums are a sign that something is wrong. Your gums should never bleed when you brush your teeth. If you experience bleeding gums, you should schedule an appointment to see your dentist. The number one cause for bleeding gums is periodontal disease. The dentist will prescribe a treatment plan.

119.   Using floss or an interdental cleaner will really make a difference. Brushing your teeth regularly is necessary but a regular toothbrush will not allow you to clean between your teeth. You should carefully clean the space between your teeth with floss or with an interdental cleaner after each meal to prevent decay.

120.   Eat an apple for your smile. Apples are a good way to clean and whiten your teeth when you cannot get to a toothbrush. When you are eating rich foods, drinking red wine, or smoking, follow it up with an apple. You will need fewer cleanings at the dentist's office if you do.

121.   Lightly brush your gums while brushing your teeth. Your gums are just as important as those choppers in your mouth. Poor care of your gums

can lead to cavities, receding gums, and even gum disease. You can really boost your dental care by paying attention to your gums much more often. A light brushing along the gum line will help keep these issues at bay.

122.   When you are brushing your teeth, make sure that you get all of the toothpaste out of your mouth by rinsing properly. Leaving toothpaste on your teeth can cause buildup, which can negatively affect the health of your mouth. After you are done, give your mouth a good rinse three times with a cup of water.

123.   Keep your toothbrush clean. Rinse it when you are done brushing, and let it dry. Use a holder for your toothbrush so that your toothbrush isn't coming into contact with things. Don't keep your toothbrush in a closed container where bacteria can grow. Get a new toothbrush every few months.

124.   Did you just break your tooth? The first thing that you need to do is get in touch with your dentist. After you get in touch with them, rinse your mouth out with warm water. Then use a cold compress on the area to reduce the swelling and decrease any pain.

125.   Little kids may be afraid to visit the dentist. Before your appointment, explain all of the wonderful things that dentists do. Choosing a pediatric dentist that makes the waiting room and exam rooms kid friendly, can really make all the difference in your child's comfort level.

126.   Visit the dentist on a regular basis. Regular dental checkups can ensure that your teeth remain strong and healthy. Your dentist is a professional, which means he or she can spot any kind of small, almost undetectable problems early, which can prevent huge problems in the future. If you do not go see a dentist regularly, minor issues will get worse and cost you a lot of money.

127.   Prior to selecting a dentist, make sure you understand what your health benefits are. Some plans will only cover certain dentists, and it is important to do your research to find out who you can and can't go to. You may wind up saving quite a bit of money as a result.

128.   To help protect your children from swallowing too much toothpaste supervise their brushing. Use only a small amount of toothpaste. Dentists generally recommend using a small pea sized amount of toothpaste for children under six years old to help protect their health. During your child's

tooth brushing routine, explain the importance of brushing each tooth properly.

129.   Use a small amount of toothpaste when you brush. While it may seem like more toothpaste would clean teeth better, it will not. The phrase, "less is more" works best when brushing your teeth. All you need is a pea-sized amount of toothpaste in the middle of your toothbrush for optimal cleaning.

130.   You can help your child overcome fears of the dentist by playing dentist together. Be the dentist and have them be a patient. Count how many teeth are in the child's mouth using a toothbrush. After you have finished, encourage your child to play dentist with a stuffed toy or doll.

131.   Although this is likely common knowledge to you, you should always brush your teeth a minimum of two times each day. However, it is important that you are brushing with a toothpaste that contains fluoride. Make sure you brush in a circular motion on each tooth, and avoid brushing too hard because this can damage your gums.

132.   When you brush your teeth can be just as important as how often you brush your teeth. Although most dentists recommend brushing twice a day, it is important to make one of those

brushings before you go to sleep at night. The production of saliva is much slower during sleep, and less saliva can allow damaging bacteria to grow.

133.   Everyone wants to have a bright, white, healthy smile, but that doesn't mean it's easy to achieve. Quitting smoking is one great stay. Another is to skip drinking coffee and red wine. The next step is to try home whitening. If that doesn't work, consider asking your dentist for a quote on their services.

134.   When you brush your teeth, make sure to brush everything inside. Your gums need to be massaged and cleaned, as does your tongue. Don't forget to rinse afterwards to ensure you get all the debris out and to also keep your breath fresh and clean for when you leave the house.

135.   Rinse your mouth out with a mixture of peroxide and water before you brush your teeth. Use half peroxide and half water to rinse your mouth out. This will help get rid of germs in your mouth. Your mouth will be more clean and your breath will be fresher.

136.   Bleeding gums are a sign that something is wrong. Your gums should never bleed when you brush your teeth. If you experience bleeding gums,

you should schedule an appointment to see your dentist. The number one cause for bleeding gums is periodontal disease. The dentist will prescribe a treatment plan.

137.   Use an electric toothbrush to brush. An electric toothbrush moves the brush head at a greater speed than what you can achieve when using a manual brush. The additional movement of the brush head cleans your teeth more effectively and with less effort. You can use your manual toothbrush when you brush between meals when not at home.

138.   It is very important to brush your teeth properly and for a long enough time. One way to make sure you are brushing thoroughly is to use an electric toothbrush. This type of brush far surpasses the manual toothbrush in the number of brush strokes per minute, so cleans much better and faster.

139.   Finding a dentist can be hard especially if you have recently moved into a new neighborhood. There are many websites available that gives dentist scores. You may also find that your primary care physician is a good source for information on dentists located in your community. Additionally, your insurance company may be able to recommend a dentist in your area.

140.   Make sure you're flossing every day. Brushing and using oral rinses can get rid of the majority of plaques, but it won't get rid of everything. Flossing allows you to ensure you're getting rid of any plaque that's gotten between your teeth. These areas can't be reached by brushing or rinsing so it's important to floss.

141.   Choose the correct toothbrush. There are different toothbrushes for children and adults, and it is important to choose the correct type. Also, be sure that the bristles aren't too hard. If the brush has an ADA seal on the box, it has been tested to ensure that the bristles won't damage your gums.

142.   If your mouth is often dry and you experience bad breath, the prescription medication you take may be the culprit. If your mouth doesn't produce enough saliva, you are more likely to end up with cavities. You should talk to your doctor about your dry mouth and ask about side effects of your medication. In most cases you can try a different medicine that does not have this side effect. If you have to stick with the same one, there may be other ways to combat a dry mouth.

143.   If you typically wear lipstick, you can actually use varieties of it to conceal tooth discoloration. Light red or medium coral shades can make teeth

look much whiter than they are. Lipstick that is lighter may have the opposite effect. If you have a bright, white smile, the lipstick may cause them to look yellow.

144.   Speak with dentists before you select one. It's important to learn about their sterilization techniques. It can affect your health, so don't forget to ask.

145.   If you are visiting your dentist for cosmetic reasons, always choose the less invasive treatments. For example is you are choosing between crowns and veneers, always opt for veneers. Veneers only require you to trim back a bit of your tooth, while crowns involve a lot more and are more damaging.

146.   Make your own toothpaste. It is very simple to do this. Simply take a bit of baking soda and mix it with a bit of water. Use the paste to brush your teeth, and then rinse your mouth completely. This is a cheaper way to get your teeth clean, and works almost as well.

147.   Studies show that following up your healthy tooth brushing habit with a fluoride rinse can reduce your chance of cavities by as much as a third! That is a lot of potential cavities, so ask your dentist to recommend the most effective wash. Pick

up a travel-size too and keep it handy for those times when you can't brush.

148.   Don't forget to take care of your gums. Your gums are a part of your mouth as well, and they affect your teeth and many other things. In fact, if you fail to take care of gum disease, it can lead to problems in your blood. Talk to your dentist about what you should do to care for your gums.

149.   Calcium plays a huge role in tooth strength, so make sure you're getting at least 500mg per day. If you're not eating a lot of dairies, nuts or calcium-rich vegetables, take a supplement instead. This is the best way to avoid enamel problems or cavities down the road, so take it seriously.

150.   Replace your non-electrical toothbrush regularly. People with electric toothbrushes should rotate their heads frequently. By using your toothbrush all the time for too long you may end up getting bacteria in your brush which then goes to your mouth. Many dentists recommend changing brushes after two or three months.

151.   Make time to clean your tongue every time that you brush your teeth. Your tongue can hold a lot of germs and needs to be kept as clean as possible. A clean tongue also promotes fresh breath. If you

want to do everything you can to have a healthy mouth you will follow this tip regularly.

152.   If you have a serious fear of the dentist and conventional methods won't work, you might want to consider taking some sort of medication. Your dentist can give you anti-anxiety medication or nitrous oxide which will make the entire dentist visit a whole lot easier. Just make sure that you don't have any adverse reactions to the medications.

153.   If your teeth are sensitive, most dentists recommend that you use a special toothpaste available at the drug store or even discount retailers to help seal up the tubules leading to the nerves in your teeth. This is the best way to deal with the problem once and for all.

154.   Replace your toothbrush every three months. The bristles on your toothbrush, no matter how much you clean them, wear out over time. They lose their cleaning effectiveness after a few months. Do yourself (and your mouth) a favor and have a replacement handy when you hit that 90 day mark.

155.   Encourage young children to brush longer by getting them fun toothbrushes. There are brushes that flash a little light with a press of a button. Have your child brush until the light automatically goes

off, usually after about two minutes. This is a fun timer for your child to use while brushing.

156.   Visit your dentist regularly. A lot of times dentists are able to spot problems before you ever have any type of pain. If they can find the problems before you have pain, they can usually fix them relatively easily. This can save you a lot of money and pain.

157.   A dental cleaner is a great way to promote dental health. Normally, inter-dental cleaners are small, disposable brushes that you can use to clean your teeth in between regular brushings. They are also helpful when cleaning between wires from braces. There are many types of this kind of brush depending on where you shop, so keep an eye out for them.

158.   You can efficiently prevent tooth decay by using a mouth wash that contains fluoride. You should check the labels of the products you buy and look for fluoride. Do not take a fluoride supplement if you decide to use some mouth wash or toothpaste that is already enriched in fluoride.

159.   In order to save tooth enamel, refrain from brushing too hard and select a soft or medium bristle toothbrush. Brushing too hard can actually

wear down tooth enamel and once the enamel is gone, it cannot be replaced! Using a hard bristle brush also can be detrimental to the enamel. Using the proper brush and technique can go a long way in preserving your tooth enamel.

160.   Make tooth brushing fun for your young children so that they will want to engage in the habit. Play games with your child like seeing who can take longest to brush their teeth. Give children stickers or stars for completing routines that include tooth brushing, and buy them a small present when they have brushed their teeth for a certain number of days in a row.

161.   Make sure that the toothpaste you use contains fluoride. While there are natural toothpastes available that do not list this as an ingredient, they do not provide the level of protection fluoride does. You have a much higher chance of developing dental issues if you use one of these brands.

162.   Finding a good dentist is important, but it is equally important to practice good oral hygiene every day. Make sure to brush your teeth in the morning and evening. Use a soft-bristled, gentle toothbrush, and brush all surfaces of each tooth. Doing this will help to keep your teeth healthy in between dental visits.

163.   Floss your teeth regularly. The importance of flossing cannot be overstated. Be sure you get between each tooth. The back teeth can be a challenge. If you are having trouble, think about using a dental pick or floss holder. There are several options available to make flossing easier.

164.   Nutrition is important to dental health. To help ensure that you are getting the necessary nutrients eat a well-balanced diet based on the USDA's food pyramid. Your diet should consist of low-fat dairy products. This will help ensure that you are getting the necessary amounts of calcium. Calcium is one of the primary building blocks of healthy teeth.

165.   Visit your dentist regularly. Many people are afraid of dentists. For the sake of your dental health, you should try your best to conquer this fear. Don't just visit your dentist when a problem arises. If you are able, try to schedule regular tooth cleanings. Regular cleanings and checkups can prevent a real problem from occurring.

166.   When brushing your teeth, make sure you are using a soft bristled toothbrush. You may be tempted to choose a medium or hard bristled brush. However, these are mush harsher on your gums and could lead to bleeding. Instead, use a soft brush and

make sure you brush your teeth for at least 2 minutes.

167.   Keep your toothbrush as clean as can be. Otherwise, you may be attracting bacteria to the bristles that then infect your mouth! Wash the bristles after every brushing, and stand your toothbrush upright so that any additional water drains down the brush. Be sure to replace your brush every few months even when you clean it well.

168.   Swollen gums and bleeding are important clues that tell you that it is time for a visit to the dentist. Bleeding gums can be caused by sensitive gums, periodontal disease, and even heart disease. Your dentist will be able to examine you so they can try and figure out why you have gums that are bleeding and swollen.

169.   Use an electric toothbrush. Not only do these brushes help keep your teeth cleaner; they are a lot of fun to use, at least compared to a normal toothbrush. This will help you make your brushing into more of a habit. Plus, they are easier to clean and will last a long time!

170.   When choosing a dentist, make sure you are able to afford his or her services. It is important that you

are aware of any upfront costs and don't get any nasty surprises after the fact. If you're unsure what the dentist charges, call or do your research online first and then make an appointment.

171.   Many people with bad breath are missing one important part of their oral hygiene process - brushing their tongue! In fact, just by brushing their tongue, people find that they quickly fix their problem and end up with fresh, clean breath in no time, so give it a try yourself!

172.   In order to keep your teeth in good shape, you should try to brush your teeth after every meal. Brushing your teeth will help to remove any food that is stuck. Brushing after meals can also help to prevent plaque from building up. If you cannot brush after after meal, try to brush at least twice a day.

173.   You should brush and clean your teeth thoroughly after every meal you have. Do not hesitate to carry a small toothbrush and some floss with you so you can clean your teeth no matter where you are. If you do not clean your teeth after a meal, make up for it by spending more time cleaning your teeth later.

174.   Remember that you are what you eat, and so are your teeth. If you smoke a lot and drink red wine often, your teeth do get discolored. If you want whiter teeth, change what you eat. If it's dark going on your mouth, your teeth are going to get dark from it.

175.   Eat as many citrus fruits as possible to keep your teeth healthy. Vitamin C helps your teeth stay strong, so you are less likely to have tooth decay if you eat plenty of oranges, lemons limes and other citrus fruits each day. However, sucking oranges or lemons can put your teeth in contact with acid that contributes to decay.

176.   Immediately brush your teeth after each meal. The longer food and debris sits on or between your teeth, the greater the chance it has to do damage. Brush within 30 minutes of your last meal for the best results. You will be glad that you did, and so will your mouth.

177.   Hydrogen peroxide has been known to help when you wish to whiten your teeth. To use hydrogen peroxide in a safe manner, pour a little into the cap and then dip a toothbrush into it. Take measures to ensure that you keep away from your gums while brushing. Rinse your mouth well, and

you can also brush your teeth with regular toothpaste aftward.

178.   Your smile can reveal your age. Misaligned or yellow teeth need to be fixed. A smile that's bad can make you look a lot older. So, if you want to look a little younger you should see a dentist to get your teeth fixed up.

179.   A good dentist can help protect your beautiful smile. When searching for a dentist, there are several good resources available to help you. Ask your primary-care doctor for a referral to a good dentist in your area. You may also want to ask your insurance carrier for recommendations of a dentist.

180.   If you think, you may have a broken jaw, do not try to handle this kind of issue yourself. The jaw will not fix itself. Take a cold compress and gently apply to the area so that swelling is reduced. Then go to the emergency room or visit your dentist immediately.

181.   One way to ensure that you do not end up with cavities is to take good care of your teeth by performing regular dental care. Brushing, flossing and using mouthwash can all help to rid your mouth of harmful bacteria. It is also an effective way to stage off cavities.

182.   If you have gum inflammation or you are susceptible to it, it is important that you avoid hot foods and drinks. These foods and beverages only cause gum inflammation and irritate problems you already have. If this is a problem for you, stick to either cool or warm foods and beverages.

183.   Stop smoking to improve your dental health. Smoking harms both teeth and gums. It can even discolor your teeth. Smoking disrupts the blood supply to the gums, which makes it harder for them to remain strong and healthy. This reduced blood supply makes it more difficult for dentists to diagnose gum diseases.

184.   Keep an eye on your gum line where you may see signs of cavities early. Your gums are where you teeth take root and where they are the most vulnerable. Many severe issues can occur here requiring root canals if they aren't taken care of early. Watch this condition and tell your dentist about changes in pain or any hint of discoloration.

185.   Sugar feeds the bad bacteria found in your mouth. To help avoid feeding the bacteria brush your teeth immediately after consuming a sugary drink or food. To help protect your mouth and increase the beneficial bacteria found in your mouth

take a probiotic supplement daily. Use both methods to increase the health of your mouth.

186.   When you have a lot of trouble with your teeth, ask your dentist about applying a sealant to your enamel. This keeps it hard and impermeable, ensuring that cavities are held at bay. The cost can be high, so ask for a quote before you get the appointment so you can afford it.

187.   The heads on your electric toothbrush must be change every two months. The bristles wear down and don't do a good job cleaning because they get too soft. Also, bacteria may build within your brush, which can actually cause your teeth to be dirtier than before.

188.   You should use some mouthwash prior to brushing. This helps to remove plaque, bacteria and food sitting against your teeth. Your brushing becomes more effective. Your teeth will be sparkly and white when you follow this tip.

189.   Make dental hygiene a priority. At a minimum, you need to be brushing your teeth twice each day. This makes sure that you get rid of food particles after eating. It also removes tooth eroding bacteria.

190.   Use a damp cloth to clean a baby's gums. This will remove any milk sugars from their gums. These sugars if left to sit, will eventually form plaque. When you wipe your baby's mouth down after feedings, you establish good oral hygiene from birth.

191.   Flossing helps remove plaque on and around your gum line and should be performed at least twice daily. When flossing, gently work the dental floss up and down between each tooth. Do not subjugate your gums to harsh flossing procedures; instead, use a gentle hand and waxed dental floss to help protect your gums.

192.   Brush ALL of your teeth, every single time. The act of brushing your teeth seems simple enough, so why do so many people do it incorrectly. A recent survey of dentists reveals that one of the most common mistakes people make is brushing only their front teeth. Don't focus on brushing only the teeth that other people see. Your molars and other back teeth are equally important, so don't neglect them!

193.   Consider asking your regular dentist about dental sealants. Sometimes brushing just isn't enough. A dental sealant is a protective coating that goes over the portions of your teeth used to chew

food. These are often put over back molars and can be very helpful in the prevention of tooth decay.

194.   If you think your teeth need to be whitened, you should schedule an appointment with your dentist. Your dentist will advise you on how to brush and floss your teeth efficiently and recommend some products you can use. In some cases, having your teeth cleaned by your dentist will be enough to make them look whiter.

195.   Although they are very healthy for your insides, acidic things like oranges and orange juice can be brutal on your teeth. The acidic properties can wear away the vital layer of enamel on the surface! Whenever you do enjoy foods high in acids, be sure and brush well as soon as possible.

196.   If you have a damaged tooth, always use tooth extraction as a last result. At the end of the day, it is always better to keep your natural teeth as opposed to choosing other, more permanent solutions. This might mean more visits to the dentists office, but you and your teeth will feel better about it.

197.   If you visit a dentist for the first time, think about how the experience was after your appointment is over. It is never to late too switch if you were not comfortable. Factors like how nice the

staff was to you and how clean the office was should all be considered.

198.   If you want your teeth to stay healthy and you enjoy having a beautiful smile, you should see your dentist every six months. Getting your teeth cleaned twice per year will help them to stay clean and free of unsightly tartar and plaque build up. Regular dental checkups are the key to preventing dental decay.

199.   Sugar feeds the bad bacteria found in your mouth. To help avoid feeding the bacteria brush your teeth immediately after consuming a sugary drink or food. To help protect your mouth and increase the beneficial bacteria found in your mouth take a probiotic supplement daily. Use both methods to increase the health of your mouth.

200.   Learn how to floss properly. Start by wrapping about 18" of floss around your middle finger. Holding that floss tightly between your fingers and thumb, gently insert around a tooth without "jamming" it in. When it reaches the gumline, gently curve it into a C-shape. Gently scrape the sides carefully. Repeat this for every tooth.

201.   Despite the fact that many popular brands of toothpaste contain baking soda, it's not something

you should be using on your teeth by itself. This will quickly erode the enamel of your teeth. This causes you to have cavities more easily and more often.

202.   Everyone wants to have a bright, white, healthy smile, but that doesn't mean it's easy to achieve. Quitting smoking is one great stay. Another is to skip drinking coffee and red wine. The next step is to try home whitening. If that doesn't work, consider asking your dentist for a quote on their services.

203.   Make sure you brush your tongue. This can be a great way to get fresh breath and to eliminate bacteria in your mouth. Just brush your tongue after you brush your teeth. Another idea is to simply get a tongue scraper, which can be more effective than a toothbrush on your tongue.

204.   A natural home remedy that can help keep your teeth clean is apple cider vinegar. This kind of vinegar provides your mouth with a number of benefits, including whitening your teeth, killing germs, and removing stains. In order for apple cider vinegar to be most effective, use it in the morning before you brush.

205.   To ensure that you get the most out of each brushing, make sure that you change your toothbrush out every three months. Bacteria can build up in the bristles over time, and by the time your toothbrush has been around for those twelve weeks, the buildup starts to counteract the good you're doing by cleaning.

206.   Fluoride supplements are a great option if you need to strengthen your teeth. Most individuals get enough fluoride by drinking mineral water and adopting a healthy diet but keep in mind that unhealthy teeth are often caused by a fluoride deficiency. Talk to your dentist if you do not know what kind of supplements you should take.

207.   It is very important to schedule dentist appointments as regularly as possible. You should see your dentist at least twice a year to have your teeth cleaned and inspected. This will help you avoid a lot of issues, adopt a better oral hygiene and allow you to save money on the long term.

208.   Believe it or not, saliva is actually your teeth's best friend! Natural saliva contains minerals, enamel-strengthening antibacterial properties and the power to neutralize acid. If you are a woman over the age of 50, menopause may be causing dry mouth, which, then leads to bad breath. Specially

formulated dry mouth products can help to eliminate embarrassing odors caused by a lack of saliva.

209.   Get a tongue scraper and use it every morning. This will clean your tongue and help remove bacteria. Your tongue will feel better and your mouth will not smell so bad. A tongue scraper is more effective than brushing your tongue with your tooth brush, and takes less time too.

210.   Eat what are known as detergent foods. These are foods that naturally clean your mouth as you eat them. Apples are the most famous example. Other choices include raw carrots, celery and popcorn. Ending a meal with a detergent food is a great way for your mouth to end the eating cleaner.

211.   It is important that you go to the dentist to have your teeth cleaned every six months. Having a professional cleaning helps to get rid of tarter build up and polishes your teeth so that they look their best. It can also help to spot cavities that might be hiding where you can't see them.

212.   You may be able to strengthen your teeth with fluoride supplements. You should take fluoride if your teeth get dark easily, or your gums are unhealthy. However, too much fluoride can put

yellow spots on your teeth. If this occurs, stop the supplements and get rid of other fluoride sources from your diet.

213.   Have your teeth checked out twice every year by a dentist. It's imperative to get your teeth cleaned. Once thoroughly cleaned, the dentist will check for gingivitis or cavities that you may need treatment. If they catch it early, they can offer simple treatments, but if not, you could need more serious procedures.

214.   Sticky foods are terrible for teeth, but that isn't just sugary gums or candies. In fact, bananas carry a ton of sugar and will stick to your teeth, leading to problems. French fries carry the same hazard, plus they come with unhealthy fats and tons of sodium. Try to avoid both if you can't brush right after eating.

215.   If you cannot afford dental work, see if your dentist will let you pay in installments. A lot of dentist offices allow people to pay for their dental work in installments in the office or with a financing company. Doing so ensures that you are able to get the help you need, when you need it.

216.   Know that some people are more prone to tarter build up than others, and not addressing this issue can be costly to your teeth. If you've learned

you have a problem with tarter, invest in a specialty toothpaste and follow it up with detailed flossing and an anti-tarter mouth wash. The effort will pay off.

217.   Make sure to visit your dentist for a cleaning every six months. Bi-annual cleanings are necessary to keep plaque under control and spot any problems before they become severe. If you have dental insurance, your cleaning visits will usually be covered at 100 percent. Keeping these appointments will save you money and headaches in the long run.

218.   Talk to your dentist about what kind of toothpaste you should use. Your dentist has a knowledge base to know what is good and what is just fancy packaging. Not only that, but your dentist can consider your particular teeth and choose one that works best for you and your lifestyle.

219.   Eat the right kinds of foods. While brushing and flossing helps you to get rid of bacteria and bits of food, eating the right foods to begin with helps too. Stay away from too many sweets, as they can start breaking down tooth enamel so that you develop cavities and other problems.

220.   When choosing a toothpaste, make sure that the product you choose includes fluoride. You can choose any flavor or brand you prefer, or you can even choose paste or gel. In fact, there are great kids options on the market which have glitter in them! That'll convince them to brush!

221.   An electric toothbrush is a great option because they offer more strokes in the same amount of time as a regular toothbrush. Electric toothbrushes can brush your teeth ten to twenty times faster than manual ones. For more strokes in less time, try an electric toothbrush.

222.   Don't skip dental appointments! Go to the dentist every six months like clockwork. If you skip even one, you could be in a world of dental hurt the next time you go. And quite often, skipping one means that you skip a few. You're health is worth your dedication to making these appointments.

223.   Kick your smoking habit. Smoking makes your teeth turn yellow, and it gives you bad, smoky breath, among other bad effects on your health. There are reported cases of mouth cancers developing in certain smokers. If you want optimal health for your teeth and gums, stay away from nicotine.

224.   Avoid using other people's toothbrushes. You may not think it's a big deal, but most people find that inappropriate. What's more, if you use someone else's toothbrush you are introducing new baceria to your mouth. That is generally something you should avoid. Therefore, make sure you only use your own toothbrush.

225.   Brush after each meal. The longer food and debris sits on or between your teeth, the greater the chance it has to do damage. If you brush within 30 minutes after eating you'll significantly limit any damage from plaque. This smart practice will help you prevent toothaches.

226.   If you want your teeth to look their best, simply brushing won't do the trick. You also have to floss your teeth regularly and use antiseptic mouthwash regularly. Mouthwash will kill more bacteria and flossing is the best way to clean the gaps between your teeth and get rid of plaque. Make sure you are brushing, flossing, and using mouthwash!

227.   Brush your teeth both in the morning and in the evening. Take your time. Many people simply go through the motions quickly and don't do an efficient job. Try timing yourself to make sure that you get your teeth very clean. If you have to, sing

the ABC song in your head, and don't stop brushing until the song is over.

228.   If you have anxiety about going to the dentist you are not alone. Many people fear the trip to the dentist, but there really is no reason to be nervous. All of the staff is highly trained and usually do their best to make sure you are comfortable, whether you are in for a simple cleaning or a complicated oral surgery.

229.   Go to dentist appointments regularly. Over time, this allows you to maintain a brighter smile with strong, healthy teeth and gums. They can spot any issues and provide useful treatment and advice to prevent more serious problems later. Without the proper dental treatment, your dental problems can become severe.

230.   Floss, floss, floss! Sure everyone brushes their teeth like they're supposed to, but how many of them actually floss. Flossing cleans the area between your teeth where food can get stuck and bacteria can spread. This will also prevent the onset of possible infections that can occur if you don't floss.

231.   Using mouthwash is a great way to clear out any loose debris and keep your breath smelling good. Make sure to avoid using a mouthwash with alcohol

in it as those brands tend to dry out the mouth, leaving a veritable wonderland for bacteria and leading to terrible problems down the road.

232.   If you are deathly afraid of spending time in the dentist's chair, you might be tempted to skip cleanings or procedures altogether. This is a bad idea, especially since poor oral hygiene can lead to gum disease or even diabetes. Consider sedation dentistry, in which the patient is not awake during the appointment. Furthermore, some dentists will prescribe sedatives prior to the appointment. If you use either option, you must have someone who can drive you to and from the appointment.

233.   Eating when you're not hungry not only adds weight, but can also increase your risk of cavities. If you snack throughout the day, you expose your teeth to more cavity-causing bacteria, sugars and acid. Thus, you should eat only when you're hungry in order to protect your dental health.

234.   If you're searching for the right dentist, check around to see what you can find out. Ask family and friends, check online reviews, and talk to patients of dentists you're considering. All of this will help you make a much better judgment call as to which dentist you're going to use in the future.

235.   Knowing how to properly brush your teeth is important. Using long horizontal strokes can cause abrasions or damage gums. It is better to use a 45 degree angle and brush in small strokes, up and down. The is will help you get into all of the cracks and crevices in your teeth.

236.   Try using a mouth rinse in your daily dental routine. A mouth rinse, along with daily brushing and flossing may boost your mouth's cleanliness. The antimicrobial rinses can reduce plaque and bacteria which may cause gum disease and gingivitis. Using rinses that contain fluoride also help to prevent or reduce tooth decay.

237.   Be careful to avoid biting any hard surfaces because you can crack the enamel on your teeth. Do not chew ice even though that may be enjoyable on a hot summer day. The ice can make your teeth brittle and the enamel can be damaged without you even being aware of it.

238.   Looking to improve your flossing skills? Try flossing with shut eyes. It may seem silly, but if you can floss effectively with your eyes shut, then you can floss in all sorts of situations. Flossing in bed, at work, and lots of other places will be much easier (and quicker).

239. Flossing picks make it simpler for kids to floss their teeth. However, learning how to floss with string floss wrapped around the fingers is better as more pressure is applied between the teeth and more debris is removed.

240. If you have a hard time remembering to brush your teeth in the mornings, put an extra toothbrush in your desk at work. Even if you don't end up brushing for the first time each day until your coffee break, or even lunch, cleaning your teeth always helps improve your dental health.

241. Bring your child along the next time you go to the dentist. This will get your child used to the dental office. Plus, your child will be able to meet the dentist, and all the people that work there, so when it's time for a visit, your child will be much more comfortable.

242. Consider using a Water Pik as part of your oral hygiene routine. The focused stream of water can effective rinse away and clean food particles between your teeth that your floss may not be able to reach. If you have trouble flossing your back teeth, a Water Pik may be the answer for you.

243. Visit your dentist regularly. A lot of times dentists are able to spot problems before you ever

have any type of pain. If they can find the problems before you have pain, they can usually fix them relatively easily. This can save you a lot of money and pain.

244.   To help whiten your teeth brush using baking soda. Baking soda is known for its disinfecting and cleaning properties. To use simply sprinkle a small amount of baking soda in your hand and dip your wet toothbrush into the baking soda. Then, gentle brush your teeth for at least two minutes.

245.   Take care when choosing a toothbrush. You will want to avoid a harder bristled brush to avoid gum irritation from harder brushing. Consider using a toothbrush that also incorporates a tongue cleaner. This can be of great use when you have had the occasion to drink beverages that stain easily.

246.   Brushing your teeth several times per day goes a long way toward preventing cavities. To help protect your teeth, brush after each meal, every morning and at bedtime. Chew some gum after eating if you can't brush your teeth.

247.   Take care of your toothbrush. After you finish cleaning your teeth, make sure you clean your toothbrush, too. Simply wash it off with water and place it in a toothbrush holder so that it is standing

up. Putting your toothbrush in a case is not advisable, because bacteria is more likely to grow that way.

248.   If you have realized that tooth brushing may not get all plaque because you can't see it, you can use a disclosing mouthwash that makes it show up so that you can brush your teeth better. The product should be used before your begin to brush. Plaque build-up will show as a bright blue or pink stain on your tooth surface. In some cases, it may take you awhile to brush away the stains. If you are in a rush, it's best to skip it until next time.

249.   Everyone brushes their teeth, but not everyone brushes their tongues. Whenever you are brushing your teeth it is also important to brush your tongue as well. There are several different bacteria that thrive on your tongue so make sure you keep your entire mouth clean by scrubbing your tongue too.

250.   When brushing, you should start out brushing your top gums and moving downward, or vice-versa. This is a good way to remove food debris from under your gums and clean them efficiently. You should scrub from side to side to some extent, but it's imperative to to brush upwards or downward from the gums as well.

251. Talk to your dentist about what kind of toothpaste you should use. Your dentist has a knowledge base to know what is good and what is just fancy packaging. Not only that, but your dentist can consider your particular teeth and choose one that works best for you and your lifestyle.

252. If you want a new dentist, you may want to call your insurance provider. You may be able to receive recommendations from your dentist. Use this list to check out every single dentist and locate the best one for you.

253. Sometimes eating certain foods is helpful after you've had a meal. In fact, eating an apple after a meal can help loosen debris from the teeth and gums and get your mouth feeling fresh again. It also can remove built up gunk from the surfaces of your teeth, plus it's low in sugar.

254. If you are thinking about getting a tongue or a lip piercing, you should know that this trend could have devastating effects on your teeth and gums. A metal piercing could crack a tooth badly and having a piercing rub on your gums constantly will cause them to become inflamed.

255. When you wake up, brush your teeth to get rid of all the accumulated debris from sleeping and

breathing through your mouth, leaving dried saliva behind. The next time to brush is just before bed, cleaning out everything you've eaten throughout the day and cleaning your mouth for the overnight hours.

256.   When flossing, gently slide the floss up and down the sides of BOTH teeth. Also, slip it beneath the gums and slide it back and forth to clear out any gunk. There are also brushes you can use which slip between the teeth and clear out anything left behind if floss doesn't do a good enough job.

257.   Before you pick out a dentist, you should make sure they're the right person for the job. Vet your dentist on the Internet by checking out his website and online reviews. Doing a bit of Internet research can help you find the dentist who is right for you. Take notes on which dentists you feel most comfortable with and make a wise final decision.

258.   Do not brush too vigorously or too often. You may think that that is helping, but the overall damage can be really devastating to your mouth. Brush three times a day for optimum results.

259.   There are things you can eat that can help your teeth. For example, eating an apple will help to clean your teeth. Broccoli, carrots and other hard

vegetables can accomplish perform the same function. Eat crunchy food regularly to help keep your teeth clean. Choose fruits and vegetables that are high in vitamin C for superb dental health.

260.   Prevention is the key to avoiding expensive dental work. Most dental problems are completely avoidable when you take preventative measures. Some important preventative measures are brushing your teeth twice daily, flossing daily, and seeing the dentist for a teeth cleaning once yearly. Avoiding sugary drinks like Kool-Aid and soft drinks will also help.

261.   You may be aware that brushing your teeth twice a day is the way to keep your teeth clean and healthy, but there are times when it is important to brush more often. If you eat certain foods with a high sugar content, you need to spend more time brushing so that you can prevent tooth decay and enamel erosion.

262.   Sugar is a major cause of most types of tooth decay. Eating sugar isn't the only problem. Drinking sugar can be even more harmful. When you drink sugary drinks, the sugary residue just sits on your teeth. It coats your mouth. As long as the sugar is on your teeth, it is causing damage.

263.   Be sure you take your time when you brush your teeth. Many people brush, but rush through it. Don't make this mistake. When you brush your teeth, take your time. Make the most of the time when your brushing your teeth. Brush for two minutes, at least.

264.   Home whitening kits are a great short-term fix for lightly stained teeth. However, many people report burning and increased sensitivity caused by the gel uses in the kits. If oral sensitivity is turning you off of home whitening, use a fluoride gel immediately before and after you apply the whitening product. Your teeth will be noticeably less sensitive.

265.   Watch around your gum line to see if there are signs of decay. The gum-line is very vulnerable and is the point at which many nerves begin. If you fail to care for them, it could mean having a root canal done. Watch your gum line for changes and if you see any, make an appointment with your dentist.

266.   Get a dental checkup ahead of your six month appointment if you are going abroad for more than a week or two. It is good to have a professional look over your mouth and teeth and make sure that you are not going to have any surprise issues while overseas.

267.   When it comes to taking care of your teeth, the best thing, you can do is brush your teeth twice a day. Most of us are good about brushing each morning, but not nearly as many people choose to brush at night. When you don't brush your teeth at night, you are allowing all the bacteria you've collected throughout the day to breed throughout the night.

268.   When you wake up, brush your teeth to get rid of all the accumulated debris from sleeping and breathing through your mouth, leaving dried saliva behind. The next time to brush is just before bed, cleaning out everything you've eaten throughout the day and cleaning your mouth for the overnight hours.

269.   Replace your toothbrush every three months. The bristles on your toothbrush, no matter how much you clean them, wear out over time. They lose their cleaning effectiveness after a few months. Do yourself (and your mouth) a favor and have a replacement handy when you hit that 90 day mark.

270.   Bleeding gums are a sign that something is wrong. Your gums should never bleed when you brush your teeth. If you experience bleeding gums, you should schedule an appointment to see your

dentist. The number one cause for bleeding gums is periodontal disease. The dentist will prescribe a treatment plan.

271.   Make dental hygiene a priority. Brush teeth twice daily every day. Brushing your teeth helps remove food particles from your teeth. Plus, the bacteria that's there will be removed in the process!

272.   Always thoroughly rinse your toothbrush after using it because the germs that you just removed from your mouth will be on the toothbrush. By rinsing it off, you will remove the germs and the remnants of old toothpaste which can build up. Follow up the rinse by tapping the toothbrush on the edge of the sink to shake excess water off of it.

273.   Never let an infection in your mouth go untreated for longer than is necessary. A mouth infection can be very serious, and can eventually lead to an infection of your blood. If you let that go to long it can reach your brain and then lead to death. While this is not common, it very well could happen.

274.   To make sure you get the most out of brushing, make sure that you don't eat any food after you brush for the night. If you are thirsty, you can drink some water. However, food or drinks with any

sugar will leave a residue on your teeth overnight, undoing much of the work you did by brushing.

275.   Jaw clenching can cause dental issues. Repeated clenching can break your teeth. Learn to recognize when you are clenching your jaw and work to stop the habit.

276.   To maintain optimal dental health, invest in two cups if you and your spouse both share the same mouthwash. If you both drink from the bottle, the bacteria in your mouths will get into the bottle and may spread to the other spouse's mouth. Having your own cup ensures that what comes out of your mouth doesn't go into anyone else's.

277.   Eat an apple for your smile. Apples are a good way to clean and whiten your teeth when you cannot get to a toothbrush. When you are eating rich foods, drinking red wine, or smoking, follow it up with an apple. You will need fewer cleanings at the dentist's office if you do.

278.   Prevention is the key to avoiding expensive dental work. Most dental problems are completely avoidable when you take preventative measures. Some important preventative measures are brushing your teeth twice daily, flossing daily, and seeing the dentist for a teeth cleaning once yearly. Avoiding

sugary drinks like Kool-Aid and soft drinks will also help.

279.   Meet with a dentist or periodontist if you notice that brushing your teeth causes you to bleed. You may have gum disease if you have bleeding gums. This can become a serious problem if not treated. Gum disease is something that can affect you by causing infections, tooth loss, diabetes, and bone loss.

280.   Eat as many citrus fruits as possible to keep your teeth healthy. Vitamin C helps your teeth stay strong, so you are less likely to have tooth decay if you eat plenty of oranges, lemons limes and other citrus fruits each day. However, sucking oranges or lemons can put your teeth in contact with acid that contributes to decay.

281.   It is important that you go to the dentist to have your teeth cleaned every six months. Having a professional cleaning helps to get rid of tarter build up and polishes your teeth so that they look their best. It can also help to spot cavities that might be hiding where you can't see them.

282.   To select the most effective mouthwash, be sure to look for alcohol-free brands. Mouthwash containing alcohol tends to dry the mouth out.

Saliva is actually beneficial to your teeth and assists in breaking down some bacteria. As saliva plays an important role in dental health, care should be taken to select mouthwash brands, which contain no alcohol, which can hinder saliva production.

283.   Are you dealing with tooth decay? You should go to your dentist and ask about dental sealant. Your dentist will be able to place a protective coating on your molars so the tooth decay does not go any further. Do not wait for the situation to get worse; go to your dentist as soon as you notice the decay.

284.   Get your children used to brushing their teeth as soon as they start to come in. Wipe infants' teeth clean with a cloth every day so they are used to putting something in their mouth to clean their teeth. When your children become toddlers, let them have a toothbrush to play with and chew on. Then, when they get a little older, show them how to brush their teeth.

285.   Sugar is a major cause of most types of tooth decay. Eating sugar isn't the only problem. Drinking sugar can be even more harmful. When you drink sugary drinks, the sugary residue just sits on your teeth. It coats your mouth. As long as the sugar is on your teeth, it is causing damage.

286. An important step in ensuring you receive quality dental care at all times is making sure to verify the licensing and credentials of any care provider you choose. Education and experience are critical to your provider's ability to give you the care and attention you need. Thus, making sure they have the expertise and background they claim to have is a key step in finding the sort of professional you deserve.

287. The health of your gums and teeth is severely compromised by using any form of tobacco product. Research how smoking can negatively effect your oral health. Your smartest move would be to quit this habit as quickly as possible. Your dentist will be able to offer some suggestions.

288. If you have young children, it is important you teach them about dental hygiene. Show them how to properly brush their teeth and teach them to recognize the foods that will damage their teeth. They will have a better hygiene as adults if they get into the habit of brushing and flossing regularly.

289. If you are thinking about getting a tongue or a lip piercing, you should know that this trend could have devastating effects on your teeth and gums. A metal piercing could crack a tooth badly and having

a piercing rub on your gums constantly will cause them to become inflamed.

290.   Chewing gum that's sugarless is a fantastic way to have strong and healthy teeth. Gum chewing will produce more saliva inside your mouth. This helps reduce cavity causing plaque on the teeth. That will also neutralize acids that erode teeth.

291.   When you brush your teeth, make sure to brush everything inside. Your gums need to be massaged and cleaned, as does your tongue. Don't forget to rinse afterwards to ensure you get all the debris out and to also keep your breath fresh and clean for when you leave the house.

292.   Use an electric toothbrush to brush. An electric toothbrush moves the brush head at a greater speed than what you can achieve when using a manual brush. The additional movement of the brush head cleans your teeth more effectively and with less effort. You can use your manual toothbrush when you brush between meals when not at home.

293.   Often overlooked, but still quite important in terms of proper dental care is the subject of nutrition. By following a well-balanced diet that is high in essential nutrients, it is easier to stave off tooth decay. By steering clear of sticky candies and

items high in processed carbohydrates, you will have an easier time keeping the surfaces of the teeth clean throughout the day.

294.   After you have brushed your teeth follow up with a good fluoride rinse. A fluoride rinse will help protect your teeth by hardening the enamel on your teeth. For the greatest benefit rinse for at least one minute. The proper procedure for rinsing is to swish the mouthwash between each tooth; then, finish with a quick rinsed to help freshen your breath.

295.   What kind of toothpaste do you use? It is best to use a toothpaste that contains fluoride. If you have issues with cavities, choose a toothpaste designed to reduce your risks of developing cavities. You can also choose a product designed for people with sensitive gums if this is your case.

296.   Teens tend to ignore dental care. Teens are very conscious about their looks, so remind them that bad breath will be the result when they don't brush or use mouthwash. This can motivate teens to take care of their mouth.

297.   Take care of your tooth brush. Rinse your tooth brush thoroughly after use. Store it in an upright position, allowing it to air dry. Try not to leave your

tooth brush in an enclosed area. This could encourage the growth of bacteria or even mold. If the cleanliness of your toothbrush is compromised, replace it immediately.

298.   Try your best to stop using tobacco products. Most people are not aware that smoking can cause gum disease, which leads to tooth loss in many. If you want to raise the chances of your teeth lasting much longer, try your best to get rid of your addiction to tobacco products.

299.   Brush all of the surfaces of your teeth. Many people think that they only need to clean the surfaces that are visible, but bacteria likes to hide on the hidden parts of teeth. These are the areas where various dental problems can occur. When you brush, make sure to brush the outside, inside, and chewing surfaces of every tooth.

300.   If you have a young child, consider asking your dentist about fluoride treatments at their six month dental visits. Fluoride treatments provide a longer lasting coat of protection to each tooth, and this protection lasts much longer than traditional toothpaste. This can help to keep cavities away and keep your child's teeth healthy.

301.   For the whitest, brightest smile possible, watch what you eat and drink. Beverages like coffee, tea and soda are notorious for depositing unsightly yellow and brown stains on the surface of your teeth. Darkly colored juices are also potential culprits, as are certain types of gravy and fruit products. If you do consume these items, brush your teeth immediately after doing so.

302.   Select a good dentist that can treat your long term problems. If this dentist cannot help you, he will probably refer you to a specialist who can. If a referral isn't an option, find a specialist who can address your dental issues.

303.   Don't forget to floss. A lot of people don't floss because they don't think it is important, but flossing is essential to good dental care. Make sure you floss before you brush, and you will see a difference in how much plaque forms. Flossing truly is a worthwhile task if you want to have healthy teeth.

304.   Though it may seem somewhat intuitive, one of the very best tips for practicing effective dental care is to brush and floss the teeth often. Brushing two times daily is a great start, but if possible, it is even better to do so after each and every meal. In this way, food residue and potential build-up do not have the chance to accumulate.

305.   Consider sealants for young children. Most of their decay is in the grooves on the biting surfaces of their back teeth. These pits are deep and are hard to reach with just basic brushing. Cavity-causing bacteria likes to hide deep within these areas. Sealants can fill in the tissues of their teeth and make their brushing more effective.

306.   Flossing your teeth is more effective if you do it at night rather than in the morning. If you wait until you wake up, all of the food stuck between your teeth has had the entire night to corrode the sides of your teeth, doing hours of damage to your dental health.

307.   If you desire fresh breath, you must brush twice daily -- including your tongue. Your tongue gathers food debris and bacteria, and when air passes over the tongue it causes an unpleasant odor or bad breath.

308.   If your teeth are crooked, you can get braces to straighten them. This procedure is usually done at a young age, but adults can also benefit from it. New techniques make it possible to wear braces that can be removed to make eating easier, and some types only need to be worn overnight.

309.   Talk to a dentist if you feel like you are clenching or grinding your teeth while sleeping. Both can lead to serious dental issues over time. Your dentist can help you through your options. This is not only good for you, but also for your significant other. Grinding your teeth can keep your loved one awake!

310.   Brushing is important, but especially important first thing in the morning and just before you go to sleep. Bacteria and plaque are the most prevalent in the morning. Your mouth dries out overnight, making it easier for bacteria and plague to thrive. Brushing at night helps to keep the plague down before you sleep.

311.   Brush after eating sticky foods. Foods like caramel and taffy can stick to the surface of your teeth. This can be very damaging to your teeth. Make sure that you thoroughly brush away the residue as soon as possible. Additionally, you may want to limit your consumption of these sorts of foods.

312.   If you are not sure which dentist to visit, talk to the people that you know. Chances are, if a family member or friend has had a good experience with a dentist, you will too. You can also speak with your

doctor or check online to find possibilities that might be suitable.

313.   Although they are very healthy for your insides, acidic things like oranges and orange juice can be brutal on your teeth. The acidic properties can wear away the vital layer of enamel on the surface! Whenever you do enjoy foods high in acids, be sure and brush well as soon as possible.

314.   Daily flossing is important to remember. Flossing eliminates that plaque and bacteria between your teeth where your toothbrush cannot get. It'll help to stimulate your gums, too. You can either floss in the morning or at night; however, just don't forget to floss.

315.   If you want whiter teeth, try to avoid eating or drinking anything that could harm your efforts. You don't want all your efforts to be in vain because you stick with the same bad habits. You will keep your bright smile if you eliminate certain foods and drinks from your diet.

316.   For the whitest, brightest smile possible, watch what you eat and drink. Beverages like coffee, tea and soda are notorious for depositing unsightly yellow and brown stains on the surface of your teeth. Darkly colored juices are also potential

culprits, as are certain types of gravy and fruit products. If you do consume these items, brush your teeth immediately after doing so.

317.   When you brush your teeth can be just as important as how often you brush your teeth. Although most dentists recommend brushing twice a day, it is important to make one of those brushings before you go to sleep at night. The production of saliva is much slower during sleep, and less saliva can allow damaging bacteria to grow.

318.   Before choosing a new dentist, ensure he's the best one for your needs. Do your research on the Internet and check out the dentist's website. It is very important you learn what education they have and what their beliefs are to make sure these all fit your needs. Find a dentist who makes you feel comfortable.

319.   If you find that your mouth and lips are dry a lot, tell your dentist about it. If you are taking medications, they may be the cause. Your dentist will be able to tell you whether your medications are causing your dry mouth, and can help you determine how you can treat it.

320.   Every two month, you should even change out the head of your electric toothbrush. The bristles

can get worn out from use and the result is decreased performance in effective brushing. In addition, bacteria can accumulate inside the brush, which can turn your toothbrush into a disgusting place for germs.

321.   You should brush your teeth twice daily. Brushing your teeth twice daily helps prevent cavities. Choose a toothpaste that contains fluoride to add an extra layer of protection against dental caries. When brushing your teeth use an up and down motion, this will help prevent damage to your gums.

322.   Though you may not have given much thought to it before, the dental care tools you have at home play a large role in your overall dental health. Make sure to use fluoridated toothpaste and a brush with soft bristles. You may even want to purchase a battery-powered toothbrush that is often more effective at eliminating plaque build-up.

323.   Teach your child to brush by modeling proper brushing yourself. Every night, stand in front of the mirror together and have him imitate the way you brush. By his observing you, your child will learn the proper brushing techniques. The same method can be applied to flossing as you model for him how to floss properly.

324.   Begin brushing your child's teeth as soon as they cut their first tooth. To help avoid accidental ingestion of fluoride, use only a pea-sized amount of toothpaste. Additionally, as soon as your little one has two teeth beside each other, it is time to begin flossing their teeth to protect against cavities.

325.   Friction from grinding your teeth at night can cause your enamel to erode. If you grind your teeth hard enough, you may find that you are at a greater risk for fracturing your teeth. So wearing a mouth guard is the best way to protect your teeth if you grind them in your sleep.

326.   Try to avoid clenching your jaws. Repeated clenching can break your teeth. So learn to be aware of when you clench your jaw and find a way to stop doing it.

327.   You should replace your toothbrush on a regular basis. Bacteria will grow on your toothbrush and you will keep transferring bacteria to your mouth if you do not replace your toothbrush regularly. Try buying a new toothbrush every eight to ten weeks. If you have a gum disease, change it more often.

328.   How you hold your toothbrush really does matter. It is ideal to point the bristles towards your

gums so that you are creating the right amount of friction. Additionally, it will help to remove anything that may have gotten in between your teeth and your gums, which will reduce your risk of gum disease.

329.   Make an annual dentist visit. You will greatly improve the health of your teeth with regular dentist appointments. It costs less to repair problems with teeth if these problems are caught early. If small problems are not treated, they can become big problems, which are much more difficult to fix. Quick and short treatments can maintain healthy teeth and a healthy wallet.

330.   When it comes to brushing your teeth, even your grip on the toothbrush can affect the end result. Hold the toothbrush at an angle when brushing your teeth. Next, move it in small circles. However, you will irritate your gum if you're brushing too roughly.

331.   Certain habits can keep you from having pearly white teeth. If you drink red wine, coffee, dark tea, dark juices or colas, don't be surprised if you have stained teeth. A good rule of thumb to remember is that if a liquid is dark, it will probably darken your teeth. One way to minimize staining of your teeth is to brush them immediately after drinking these dark

beverages. If you are at a location where it is not feasible for you to immediately brush, eating an apple can help you clean your teeth until you can brush them properly.

332.   You should not purchase a toothpaste advertised as a product that can whiten your teeth without checking the label first. Look for fluoride. This ingredient is absolutely necessary for healthy teeth, and some whitening toothpaste do not even contain fluoride. Try a toothpaste for a few weeks and switch to a different brand if you are not happy with the results.

333.   If you are having a difficult time paying for necessary dental work, consider visiting a dental college. College students in the later stages of their training need real people to work on, and they will often perform work at a significantly reduced cost. All students are supervised by their professors or certified dentists, so you remain in safe hands during your procedure.

334.   Some people incorrectly assume that the higher price a dentist charges, the better he or she must be. This is not the best way to determine which dentist is your best bet. The best way to find out which dentists are the most skilled, accommodating and effective is to seek recommendations and reviews.

Ask friends and family members for feedback on dentists, or search online for more information.

335.   If you are having dental issues, go the dentist right away, even if you are off your visit cycle. It may be tempting to think it's best to hold off til your normal visit, but your teeth will only be getting worse during the wait time. It may cost a few extra dollars now, but it's well worth it to keep the big dental bills away.

336.   The first mistake that people make in dental care is to buy the wrong toothbrush. You should choose a toothbrush that fits well in your mouth and reaches all areas. Your toothbrush should also fit well in your hand. If you lose your grip on your toothbrush, you could actually injure yourself.

337.   Floss every night at the minimum. And if you are serious about your dental health, floss in the morning as well. Foods get caught in your teeth and gums, and often your toothbrush won't be enough to remove the pieces. Flossing is an essential for the best dental health care possible.

338.   When you are brushing, handle the brush gently in your mouth. Proper brushing doesn't involve a lot of pressure on your teeth. You may think you are cleaning better with some pressure, but really

you are just traumatizing your gum area in the process. This can lead to receding gums and pockets.

339.   With three simple steps, you can have a healthy mouth. First of all, it is important to brush your teeth on a daily basis. To clean teeth in areas where your toothbrush can not reach, use dental floss every day. The third step in to visit your dentist regularly. It is commonly recommended to see your dentist at least twice a year.

340.   If you are considering whitening your teeth at home, you should consult your dentist first. Your dentist may be able to whiten your teeth just with a good cleaning. Your dentist should also be able to recommend at home whitening kits that should work for you. Your dentist will also be able to give you an idea of how white your teeth will be after whitening them.

341.   Make sure to see the dentist at least twice every year. Even if you only have your teeth cleaned, the hygienist will note any developing problems and point them out to the dentist. It is much easier, and cheaper too, to have any small cavities fixed before they get any bigger.

342. Always thoroughly rinse your toothbrush after using it because the germs that you just removed from your mouth will be on the toothbrush. By rinsing it off, you will remove the germs and the remnants of old toothpaste which can build up. Follow up the rinse by tapping the toothbrush on the edge of the sink to shake excess water off of it.

343. Make sure to replace your toothbrush on a regular basis. Usually a toothbrush should be replaced after three months. But you should replace it sooner if it becoming worn, falling apart or the bristles are bent out of shape. Some toothbrushes even come with color indicators that fade over time and let you know when it is time to be replaced.